ADHD POSITIVE PARENTING FOR BOYS AND GIRLS

Early Signs of ADHD Every Parent Should Know, How to Motivate Your Child, Stop Procrastination, Improve Their Focus, And Help Your Child Develop Better.

Sharon Daven

Please note the information contained within this document is for educational and entertainment purposes only. All effort has been executed to present accurate, up to date, and reliable, complete information. No warranties of any kind are declared or implied. Readers acknowledge that the author is not engaging in the rendering of legal, financial, medical or professional advice. The content within this book has been derived from various sources. Please consult a licensed professional before attempting any techniques outlined in this book.

By reading this document, the reader agrees that under no circumstances is the author responsible for any losses, direct or indirect, which are incurred as a result of the use of the information contained within this document, including, but not limited to, — errors, omissions, or inaccuracies.

Your Free Gift

As a way of saying thanks for your purchase, I'm offering this book ***BABY SAFETY TIPS*** for **FREE** to my readers.

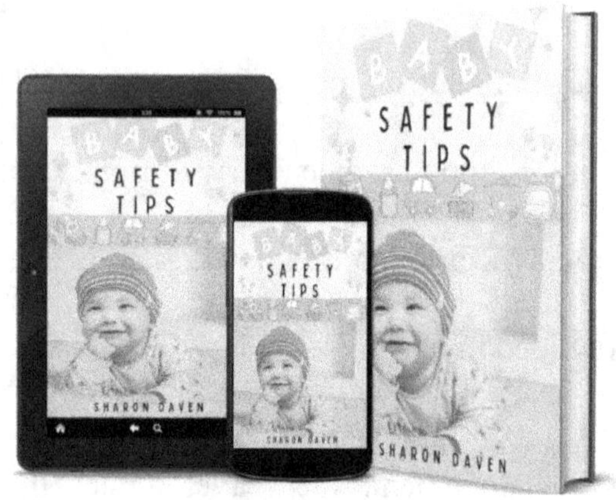

To get instant access **SCAN THE QR CODE:**

<u>**Inside this book, you will discover:**</u>

- 12-Must have products that will keep your child safe around the home

- Traveling with a baby checklist.

- How to reduce the risk of poisoning in your household.

- Toy Safety Tips.

- Safe bedding practices for infants

If you want to know how to keep your baby safe, make sure to grab this **FREE** book now.

Table of Contents

INTRODUCTION

"We do not need to cure neurodiversity. We need to embrace it."

Jonathan Mooney

Have you ever wondered why children sometimes seem out of control? They may fuss over little things; gallop about in constant motion, thump into stuff, and throw fits of tantrums. At other times, they may seem out and away, unapologetically lost in the fantasy of their own world.

While many children observe these behaviors occasionally, some go on to show these signs on a frequent note. Sensitive parents who are quick to take precautions against these recurrent patterns begin to hunt for what might be wrong or out of place preventing their kids from living a normal life. And in the quest for solution and relief, parents often find themselves in and out of health offices seeking genuine and lasting help for their wards.

Whether fear or stress is the motivation for seeking help isn't the question here. Instead, the focus is if at the end of their investigations, parents are better inclined and have achieved a level of insight needed to tackle the mission for which they set off in the first place—making their child better off.

Imagine a family that recently moved from Florida to Germany with their five-year old. Within the first year of settling into the new environment, the grown-ups soon discover that their kid lacked major English vocabularies for expressing everyday interactions which was previously not the case.

They noticed her lax, quiet, and withdrawn stance on several occasions. They couldn't argue that was her nature right from time but for some strange reason they felt something but can't seem to place their fingers on it. Was their daughter's challenge as a result of transitioning from a familiar to an unfamiliar location? Or was it based on switching from language codes from a known language to an unknown one?

They would never know until the intervention of the pediatrician who confirmed their conjectures, noting the incident as a language loss situation coupled with the offshoot of an existing neurodevelopmental disorder. It happened that the now six-year-old child had an undiagnosed case of Attention Deficit Disorder (ADD), a type of Attention Deficit Hyperactive Disorder (ADHD) that had remained hidden until that very moment.

What's Your First Response?

A study from 2011 to 2013 revealed that 9.5% of U.S. children within the age bracket of 4–17 years had been diagnosed with ADHD at one point or another. In speaking with over one hundred and fifty parents of autistic and neurodiverse children, I have understood one key behavior. I realized that a higher percentage of parents first react to the news of raising a neurodiverse child with panic. This initial reaction mostly develops because parents have zero preparation on how to handle such special cases.

I guess they're not alone anyway. After my son got diagnosed of autism fifteen years back, I remember feeling blank and muttering "How do I go forward from here?" The urgent need to see my son thrive despite the odds and my motherly instincts to be the best mother to my new born kicked me into life-long research on how to nurture and give my baby a better chance at life.

This decision has helped me to dig out practical frameworks for a model parenting of not just my fifteen-year-old autistic son or my five-year-old ADHD grandson, but also many other sons and daughters of parents who lead a similar lifestyle with their children.

How I See This Book

Once I found out the excuse for the negative reactions from many parents, it occurred to me that something can be done. Through extensive research and relentless first-hand experience, I reached an outcome that will later combat every "what-ifs" reserved in the minds of most parents and transform them to a positive "even-if" condition. In such a way, rather than asking—

- *What if I can't do anything to help my kid?*

- *What if my child starts having problems at school and I'm not there to help?*

- *What if my children don't behave like other kids their age?*

Parents can move past these panic-riddled questions to asking ones that'll inject panacea and offer immediate help like:

- *Now that I'm aware of my child's state, what other common symptoms can I look out for?*

- *What are the abnormal signs to watch out for?*

- *Is there a way to treat this condition and salvage my child's future?*

While the various neurodevelopmental conditions have no direct cure, there's how to treat and manage it. This book is a compendium of my years of extensive research, expert consultations, and personal experiences. I have organized my findings into packets of wisdom in forms of chapters and paragraphs to enlighten you on the topic of Attention Deficit Hyperactive Disorder (ADHD).

By now, you are well aware of the story surrounding my motivation for being a neurodivergent specialist. With up to five years of professionally helping parents simplify the parenting journey of their neuro-diverse children, *Autism Positive Parenting* is my first book tailored to suit the purposes of my work.

How You Should View This Book

Having this book in your hands means possessing a pool of experience where you can always draw practical advice and suggestions relating to your ADHD child. See *ADHD Positive Parenting for Boys and Girls* as an orientation tool that captures the essential aspects of dealing with your special child and offers a dimension of pure love flowing from a caring mother and concerned grandmother.

I have designed this book in two parts that spells out the nitty-gritty of ADHD in a way that allows you to have a working knowledge about the subject. In Part I, you'll learn about what ADHD really is (Chapter 1), the early signs of ADHD and how it manifests (Chapter 2), the common challenges that accompany parenting your ADHD child (Chapter 3).

Part II provides you with strategies to help your child manage ADHD (Chapter 4). You will explore the various ways involved in setting the pace for your child's happiness (Chapter 5) and finally access the best medication and method to treat ADHD.

You're now ready to debunk the myths masking ADHD and set the records straight by becoming the kind of parent that your child truly needs. View this book as the missing link between the life you visualize for your kid and that which currently obtains. Hence, you can participate in your child's life and strike satisfaction as you do.

Through the relevant stories and illustrations lined up on the pages, you are sure to find inspiration to forge forward and own your journey. And likewise, you'll find pleasure in empowering your child to embrace their journey and make their lives count.

CHAPTER ONE

ADHD: WHAT IS IT, REALLY?

"It is not uncommon for children (and adults) to receive multiple diagnoses or be misdiagnosed at first." - First Psychology

Mention ADHD anywhere in the world today and I can assure you of a catalog of conflicting thoughts reinforced in the minds of your listeners. For many, the initial train of thought may go in this format: ADHD is a title for sick or abnormal human beings. Others may think of it as a disease passed from a parent's gene to a newborn. Some might regard it as some form of unlucky accident that probably occurred to deteriorate adult life.

The possibilities that could skim through the mind upon hearing ADHD are limitless, especially for non-experts in the field. If there'll be anyone in the bulk of listeners to have a clear-cut idea of the acronym, I bet such a person must have had a past affiliation with the subject or they're probably experts in the area.

In this chapter, my focus will be to reveal the fine line that separates the amateurs from the professionals. What do the experts know that places them a cut above the rest when talking about ADHD? Can anyone dig into the roots of this subject or is it an oasis only reserved for gurus in psycholinguistics, neurology, social workers, or medical practitioners?

No doubts, professionals who diagnose and treat ADHD are hard wired to know the subject brick by brick, layer by layer. But the sweet spot is they hold no autonomy on who should know what when it comes to having a working knowledge of either ADHD or any other neurodevelopmental disorder.

Essentially, what you and I who never had school knowledge about ADHD need is not always full-blown facts but a foundational awareness upon which we can build on later. During my years of diving deep into aspects of research about neurodiversity, I have uncovered well past just basics. More than that, I have compared, contrasted, tested, and applied my findings to real life situations and they worked. In giving a robust explanation of the meaning of ADHD, I'll be calling on some of my first-hand experiences and also testimonials of people facing the struggle on a real-time basis.

What experts know about ADHD

ADHD is an acronym that stands for attention-deficit/hyperactivity disorder. It is a "neurodevelopmental disorder (NDD) presenting with inattention, hyperactivity, and impulsivity." In other words, it is a brain condition that makes it almost impossible for children to control their behavior. It affects millions of children and often persists throughout their lifetime.

Most people struggling with ADHD as adults have had it since they were children but they weren't diagnosed with it as a child. This scenario is prevalent because ADHD is difficult to diagnose in children less than six years of age. Yet, it is the most common disorder affecting children. An estimated 8.4% of children and 2.5% of adults are diagnosed of ADHD.

The disorder is noted to be more popular in boys than in girls. Research known as the European ADORE study which stretched through the period of 24 months and spreading across 10

European countries investigated children and teenagers within the ages of 6-18 years. Out of a total number of 1478 children the result showed that a whopping 84.3% of the group (1222 participants) were boys while the girls took the smaller percentage of 15.7 (231).

In taking note of visible signs and symptoms that accompany ADHD, I call to mind the criteria established by the American Psychiatric Association (APA 1994): the patient needs to exhibit behaviors related to inattention (for example, may fail five close attentions to details or may make careless mistakes in school work or other tasks), hyperactivity or impulsivity (they may fidget with objects, tap their hands, and shake their feet excessively).

Many children may have a hard time sitting still, waiting for their turn, or paying attention. In classrooms and teaching centers, these behaviors are unlikely to be about disobedience or defiance. Precisely, it needs to be regarded as a form of natural tendency in likely situations. As a matter of fact, some adults with ADHD must express such repetitive actions to gain knowledge and get things under control at work.

APA (1994) in discussing the symptoms associated with ADHD pointed out that such symptom must be in play for six months at least, inconsistent with developmental level, impair social or academic functioning, present before age seven, and must have been identified in two or more settings (including the home and school).

Taking a step further to review the propositions of the Diagnostic and Statistical Manual of Mental Disorder (DSM-5), these paragraphs highlight the characteristics of a child with ADHD:

A. A persistent pattern of inattention and/or hyperactivity-impulsivity that interferes with functioning or development, as characterized by (1) and/or (2):

1. Inattention

2. Hyperactivity and impulsivity

B. Several inattentive or hyperactive-impulsive symptoms were present prior to age 12 years.

C. Several inattentive or hyperactive-impulsive symptoms are present in two or more settings (e.g., at home, school, or work; with friends or relatives; in other activities).

D. There is clear evidence that the symptoms interfere with, or reduce the quality of, social, academic, or occupational functioning.

E. The symptoms do not occur exclusively during the course of schizophrenia or another psychotic disorder and are not better explained by another mental disorder (e.g., mood disorder, anxiety disorder, dissociative disorder, personality disorder, substance intoxication or withdrawal).

Oftentimes, the disorder is prevalent in children during elementary school but the symptoms may rescind as the child grows into adolescence and adulthood. However, the difficulties with restlessness, inattention, poor planning, and impulsivity persist, which form the core types of ADHD disorder as I will explain shortly.

Types of ADHD

Even as there are various developmental and behavioral disorders that may materialize in children including the emotional-obsessive-compulsive disorder (OCD), conduct disorder (CD), autism spectrum disorder (ASD), and oppositional defiant disorder (ODD), the visible signs and symptoms to look out for in an ADHD child is unmistaken. A close look at the three types of ADHD will provide insights for the specifications to look out for in diagnosing ADHD.

The 3 types of ADHD are predominantly inattentive presentation, predominantly hyperactive/impulsive presentation, and combined presentation.

1. Predominantly Inattentive Presentation

Children that have this form of ADHD are not overly active. Inattentive unveil itself with challenges that relate to staying on tasks, finishing tasks, focusing, and organizing. Since children with this type of ADHD rarely disrupt class activities, their symptoms may be subtle but still quite noticeable. Some studies have it that this type is more common with girls that have ADHD than boys. Here's the bottom line: children might not necessarily display all the symptoms for diagnosis to be made. Six or five (for individuals who are 17 years and older) of the following symptoms occur frequently (according to DSM-5):

a. Often fails to give close attention to details or makes careless mistakes in schoolwork, at work, or during other activities (e.g., overlooks or misses details, work is inaccurate).

b. Often has difficulty sustaining attention in tasks or play activities (e.g., has difficulty remaining focused during lectures, conversations, or lengthy reading).

c. Often does not seem to listen when spoken to directly (e.g., mind seems elsewhere, even in the absence of any obvious distraction).

d. Often does not follow through on instructions and fails to finish schoolwork, chores, or duties in the workplace (e.g., starts tasks but quickly loses focus and is easily sidetracked).

e. Often has difficulty organizing tasks and activities (e.g., difficulty managing sequential tasks; difficulty keeping materials and belongings in order; messy, disorganized work; has poor time management; fails to meet deadlines).

f. Often avoids, dislikes, or is reluctant to engage in tasks that require sustained mental effort (e.g., schoolwork or homework; for older adolescents and adults, preparing reports, completing forms, reviewing lengthy papers).

g. Often loses things necessary for tasks or activities (e.g., school materials, pencils, books, tools, wallets, keys, paperwork, eyeglasses, mobile telephones.

h. Is often easily distracted by extraneous stimuli (for older adolescents and adults, may include unrelated thoughts).

i. Is often forgetful in daily activities (e.g., doing chores, running errands; for older adolescents and adults, returning calls, paying bills, keeping appointments).

2. Predominantly hyperactive/impulsive presentation

Hyperactivity means excessive movement or energy like fidgeting, inability to sit still, and talkativeness. Meanwhile, impulsivity refers to making decisions and taking actions without thinking about the consequences though. Children with this kind of ADHD show both of the qualities but can pay attention despite all. This group is the least common. Again, children in these categories might not necessarily display all the symptoms for diagnosis to be made. Six or five (for individuals who are 17 years and older) of the symptoms occur frequently (according to DSM-5):

a. Often fidgets with or taps hands or feet or squirms in their seat.

b. Often leaves a seat in situations when remaining seated is expected (e.g., leaves his or her place in the classroom, in the office or other workplace, or in other situations that require remaining in place).

c. Often runs about or climbs in situations where it is inappropriate. (Note: In adolescents or adults, may be limited to feeling restless.)

d. Often unable to play or engage in leisure activities quietly.

e. Is often "on the go," acting as if "driven by a motor" (e.g., is unable to be or uncomfortable being still for extended time, as in restaurants, meetings; may be experienced by others as being restless or difficult to keep up with).

f. Often talks excessively.

g. Often blurts out an answer before a question has been completed (e.g., completes people's sentences; cannot wait for a turn in conversation).

h. Often has difficulty waiting his or her turn (e.g., while waiting in line).

i. Often interrupts or intrudes on others (e.g., butts into conversations, games, or activities; may start using other people's things without asking or receiving permission; for adolescents and adults, may intrude into or take over what others are doing).

3. Combined Presentation

This occurs when the characteristics of both the inattentive and hyperactive/impulsive type of ADHD materializes in the individual. Although ADHD isn't a spectrum condition, the diverse groups in which it exists offers different layers that make the experience of each ADHD child unique in its way. For instance, a family having two children with ADHD might find it wise to deal with each child separately. Why is that? Just as every human being is unique and our brains work differently, in the same vein, every ADHD child is unique with brains wired differently. No two ADHD persons are the same.

Edward M. Hallowell, an American psychiatrist, was diagnosed with ADHD himself. And he describes having ADHD as having "a race-car brain with bicycle brakes." He goes on to express how almost impossible it is for others to understand how it feels to have ADHD. It's like having "a mélange of often contradictory tendencies and traits that swirl around within you," he continues, "stirring up different parts of your life at different times as it makes its inconsistent rounds."

Founder of the Hybrid Shop Matt Curry became diagnosed with ADHD in 1978 in his seventh grade. To assuage his disorders, he was prescribed Ritalin but after a solid year of taking the medication, his parents and doctors felt it would be great to discontinue it. Eureka! Curry discovered that he could succeed without treating ADHD.

Curry completed his school and off he went working in automobile stores, doing amazingly well at each of his work places he proceeded to start his own auto repair shop. From his one shop he quickly grew to ten, rising as the owner of the largest independent auto-repair chains in Washington, D.C. His story soon birthed a book which he titled, The A.D.D. helping thousands of entrepreneurs to grow their business too. Curry is famous for this quote where he spells out that: "ADHD is my superpower. I'm successful because of it, not in spite of it." In his story, he tells of how when a million ideas run through his mind, he records them on a whiteboard and cuts them down to "three things I need to do." He breaks down each of the three things into what he calls the vision, the game plan, and the message which translates as what he wants to do, how, and why.

The story of actress Jessica McCabe stands contrary to that of Curry when she decided to let go of her ADHD medication. McCabe was diagnosed with ADHD at 12 and kicked off her medication intake as soon as possible. As she matured, Jessica decided to stop medication as she thought she no longer needed it. For eighteen months she paused, but "that was a bad idea" she said. Starting a new and different medication certainly helped although she still battled ADHD symptoms.

Jessica witnessed a turn of the tides in her early thirties while still waiting tables, struggling with her acting career, and counting several failed relationships. It was at that moment she discovered that meds were never the answer to all symptoms. By starting her Youtube Channel "How to ADHD" where she shared tools and tips that might help her and her audience, she filled the void within her. Today, McCabe continues to take medication for ADHD coupled with her daily usage of fidget toys and leading a system that helps others live better with ADHD. That's how she makes meaning with her lifestyle.

What Causes ADHD?

Scientists, psychologists, physicians, and educators have reached a consensus that ADHD is a genetically influenced, neurologically based disorder. Little wonder this has given rise to studies about the anatomy of the brain of ADHD patients and genetics. Specific genes are believed to aid the dysfunction of the frontal lobes in the cerebral cortex and their connection to subcortical structures in the limbic system and the cerebellum.

The prefrontal cortex which is sometimes referred to as the executive part of the brain could be affected by environmental factors such as injuries sustained before, during, or after birth mostly caused by infection, physical trauma, or lack of oxygen at birth. Kahn (et al. 2003) revealed that in one study, children exposed to prenatal smoking and homozygous for the DAT1 10-repeat allele were at extremely increased risk of hyperactivity, impulsivity, and oppositional symptoms, while neither factor alone was linked significantly.

Also, evidence exposes that there's a large genetic component to ADHD even if no specific gene has been recognized to cause ADHD. A child diagnosed with ADHD likely points out that siblings, parents, or grandparents have shown the symptoms. Most times, a diagnosis in one child within a family lead to several others in the same family. Thus, indicating that ADHD is highly heritable.

Also, there can be an imbalance in neurotransmitters. That is, the 'chemical messengers' in the brain that are underlying our emotions, reactions, and other related mechanisms. It should be noted that the 'imbalances' are not unique to ADHD but can play a part in many other conditions.

Other research has suggested that children with ADHD have smaller certain brain regions compared to peers. Yet, this difference in size ceases to exist overtime and by 16 to 18 years of age, young people's brains would have come to develop those regions too. The possibilities of some developmental delays are still rampant and can impart on their life at school or home.

Brain images are often treated like "neurological fingerprints: indelible and intractable." And when brain imaging maps out the differences in the way a child's brain functions, people generally assume that these differences are inherent and unchanging rather than an influence of environmental conditions.

What is solidly guaranteed, however, is that ADHD doesn't result due to poor parenting as some wrongly admit. And a child showing ADHD symptoms isn't motivated to do so simply because of their 'bad character.' Instead, the words of New York Psychiatrist Esther Wender sum it up when she said:"(ADHD) is identified by a cluster of typical behaviors and has no definitive biological maker. And because the condition cannot be objectively defined, the decision to treat will also be based on diagnostic uncertainties. The published diagnostic criteria lend an aura of objectivity to the diagnosis, but the application of these criteria is based on subjective judgments regarding the accuracy of information given by parents and teachers."

ADHD: Self-Diagnosis or Clinical Diagnosis?

There's no single test for ADHD – no blood, brain, or psychological examination that can ascertain that a person has the condition. Usually, clinicians and caregivers work hand-in-hand to assess and diagnose ADHD in a child. The parents can observe the specific symptoms in the child as highlighted above, especially when it lasts and outlasts the six months ultimatum period.

Three categories of caregiver's matter when it comes to offering feedback for the purpose of diagnosis. They are: parents and grandparents, school teachers, and other caregivers like sports team leader, scout leader and the like. It is preferable to involve them during the diagnosis stage because they need to put in much work later in helping to correct the disorder in the child in the long run.

How ADHD is diagnosed

In bringing the existence of ADHD in a child to light, clinicians often suggest a variety of steps and assessments that span across several life areas to help determine the presence or absence in a child. These can include:

- Interviews with parents and other caregivers to have a grip on the child's development and behavior and get the big picture of what is going on in the family at large

- Interviews with the ADHD patient who has come of age to understand their perspective on what they're struggling with.

- Observing the child's behaviors in different situations across diverse settings

- Using questionnaires and psychological assessments to look at various areas of functioning –reading skills, arithmetic skills, etc.

- Further probing through clinical examination to exclude any underlying medical and neurological issues that could explain the problems the individual faces

The next image represents an example of an ADHD clinician questionnaire/ass

NICHQ Vanderbilt Assessment Scale—PARENT Informant

Today's Date: __________ Child's Name: __________________________________ Date of Birth: __________

Parent's Name: _______________________________________ Parent's Phone Number: __________

Directions: Each rating should be considered in the context of what is appropriate for the age of your child. When completing this form, please think about your child's behaviors in the past **6 months.**

Is this evaluation based on a time when the child ☐ was on medication ☐ was not on medication ☐ not sure?

Symptoms	Never	Occasionally	Often	Very Often
1. Does not pay attention to details or makes careless mistakes with, for example, homework	0	1	2	3
2. Has difficulty keeping attention to what needs to be done	0	1	2	3
3. Does not seem to listen when spoken to directly	0	1	2	3
4. Does not follow through when given directions and fails to finish activities (not due to refusal or failure to understand)	0	1	2	3
5. Has difficulty organizing tasks and activities	0	1	2	3
6. Avoids, dislikes, or does not want to start tasks that require ongoing mental effort	0	1	2	3
7. Loses things necessary for tasks or activities (toys, assignments, pencils, or books)	0	1	2	3
8. Is easily distracted by noises or other stimuli	0	1	2	3
9. Is forgetful in daily activities	0	1	2	3
10. Fidgets with hands or feet or squirms in seat	0	1	2	3
11. Leaves seat when remaining seated is expected	0	1	2	3
12. Runs about or climbs too much when remaining seated is expected	0	1	2	3
13. Has difficulty playing or beginning quiet play activities	0	1	2	3
14. Is "on the go" or often acts as if "driven by a motor"	0	1	2	3
15. Talks too much	0	1	2	3
16. Blurts out answers before questions have been completed	0	1	2	3
17. Has difficulty waiting his or her turn	0	1	2	3
18. Interrupts or intrudes in on others' conversations and/or activities	0	1	2	3
19. Argues with adults	0	1	2	3
20. Loses temper	0	1	2	3
21. Actively defies or refuses to go along with adults' requests or rules	0	1	2	3
22. Deliberately annoys people	0	1	2	3
23. Blames others for his or her mistakes or misbehaviors	0	1	2	3
24. Is touchy or easily annoyed by others	0	1	2	3
25. Is angry or resentful	0	1	2	3
26. Is spiteful and wants to get even	0	1	2	3
27. Bullies, threatens, or intimidates others	0	1	2	3
28. Starts physical fights	0	1	2	3
29. Lies to get out of trouble or to avoid obligations (ie, "cons" others)	0	1	2	3
30. Is truant from school (skips school) without permission	0	1	2	3
31. Is physically cruel to people	0	1	2	3
32. Has stolen things that have value	0	1	2	3

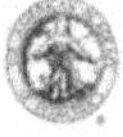

American Academy of Pediatrics

DEDICATED TO THE HEALTH OF ALL CHILDREN™

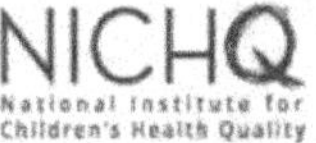

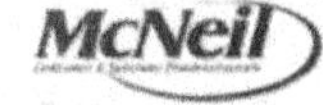

It is vital to note that other conditions can resemble ADHD in particular aspects including cases of Asperger's or autism. But a multiple diagnosis will help to split the difference and also filter ADHD from other comorbid conditions.

It is vital to note that other conditions can resemble ADHD in particular aspects including cases of Asperger's or autism. But multiple diagnosis will help to split the difference and also filter ADHD from other comorbid conditions. People will often have two or more conditions occurring simultaneously and they're called comorbid conditions. For instance, some common ones with ADHD are

- Autism Spectrum Conditions (ASC) and ADHD

- Dyslexia and ADHD

- ADHD and anxiety.

Historically, many doctors believed that comorbid situations were impossible but, it has been proven that many individuals with one condition also have traits of another.

As I attempt to close this chapter, I'll like to debunk some other erroneous ideas about ADHD that people might have assumed with no proof. By laying bare what really holds true about the subject, you will find out what constitutes the scope of ADHD and what doesn't.

5 Main Myths about ADHD

1: ADHD isn't a real medical condition

Research posits that ADHD is hereditary and medical imaging attest to the fact there's a difference between the brain development of ADHD and typical people. Many would generally assume that ADHD is only a problem of motivation and laziness on the part of the patient who need to push themselves and try harder. All lies.

Fact: The National Institutes of Health, the Centers for Disease Control and Prevention, and the American Psychiatric Association all recognize ADHD as a medical condition. ADHD is regarded as the most common childhood conditions.

2: Only boys have ADHD

This idea likely sprung up by having half knowledge of what ADHD really is. Up to date, many have no insight about the types of ADHD we have but only base judgment on what meets the eye. Symptoms categorized under the Hyperactive/Impulsive presentation are the quickest to recognize and this must have formed the foundation for this misbelief.

Fact: Yes, boys are much more diagnosed of ADHD than girls. But that doesn't cancel the fact that girls have it too. In many instances, boys are diagnosed with the Hyperactive/Impulsive presentation while the inattentive type is common with girls.

3: ADHD is a learning disability

The truth is, ADHD children need to get help in school and this has translated to the presence of learning disability in most people's minds.

Fact: ADHD isn't a learning disability. While it can hinder learning, it doesn't cause difficulty in specific skills like reading, writing, or arithmetic. However, the comorbid conditions that occur with ADHD may have contributed to the thought that ADHD is a disability.

4: ADHD has no treatment

It makes sense for people to think that ADHD has no treatment but sooner than later, an ADHD patient will definitely outgrow it. Makes sense but not true.

Fact: There's no known cure for ADHD but treatment is possible. Symptoms may lessen or fade away as kids get older but they don't totally outgrow ADHD.

5: ADHD is 'bad behavior' caused by 'bad parenting'

Come to think of it. The symptoms of ADHD do look like the impart of poor parenting on a child. The various uncontrolled behaviors bear semblance with indiscipline. But that isn't the case with ADHD.

Fact: Fidgeting, display of excessive energy, and being impulsive are signs of a medical condition and never the lack of a good and proper upbringing.

In the next chapter I will describe how ADHD manifests in boys and girls. Studying these intricate and particular symptoms will help you to spot if your child is showing early signs of the condition and thus can take action or if in fact the symptoms have no connection with ADHD you can dismiss it in your heart.

KEY TAKEAWAY:

- ADHD is a genetically influenced, neurologically based disorder that makes it almost impossible for children to control their behavior.

- The 3 types of ADHD are predominantly inattentive presentation, predominantly hyperactive/impulsive presentation, and combined presentation.

- There's no single test for ADHD to ascertain that a person has the condition. Parents work hand in hand with clinicians and caregivers to observe and diagnose likely ADHD symptoms.

- ADHD is not due to bad parenting but a real medical condition that has a treatment but no cure.

CHAPTER TWO

HOW ADHD MANIFESTS:

EARLY SIGNS IN A CHILD

"It's not just about Asperger's and autism (or ADHD) – all of our brains are different" - Reitman Hackie

I exposed you to the basic knowledge of ADHD in the last chapter. You learned about the types, causes, and the best way to diagnose and recognize ADHD symptoms. Also, the erroneous myths about ADHD were debunked and decentralized from what really holds true when experts discuss the disorder.

Pretty much I could start to call you an expert now if not for the official need of a certification. But if you ask me, I'll say every parent who continues to deal with an ADHD child from childhood through teenage hood to adulthood must have mastered this behavioral pattern they have witnessed in their child for years now.

More or less, you have wielded a form of power that comes with experience and have become increasingly capable of managing the excesses that may unfold in the events of your child's life. I know this because I've been on that road myself and I'm still right on track. Through my journey as a mother of an autistic child and grandmother of a five-year-old ADHD child, I have found this wild passion to understand and help my child and grandchild maximize all of their potential even while living with disorders.

This sacred vision comes alive each time I meet with concerned parents who desire nothing but for their kid to have the best of life regardless of the limitations. I strongly resonate with this as I sit listening to the parents of ADHD kids pour their hearts out about receiving adequate help for their kids.

One of the many cases that rings in my memory is that of Daniel's parents. I will never forget that afternoon when a man in his thirties walked into my shelved office with a squint in his eyes. It was hard to tell if he was trying to get accustomed to the drab ambiance of my office as opposed to the scorching sun outside.

Closely walking behind, him was a woman with brisk gaits grabbing onto a limp-haired child that would be about four to five years old. Wide-eyed and frequent smiles interrupted by blank stares and fixed gazes. His activities gave me a clue to work with even before the grown-ups opened their mouths to speak.

From what I discovered; Daniel wasn't their direct child but the husband's nephew who's now in their custody after both his parents lost their lives in a car accident two months back. Luke and his wife Rita had volunteered to raise the child and see to it that he fulfilled all of his dreams and lacked nothing.

But the latest developments of Daniel's erratic behaviors might just be starting to cause an uproar that would lead the young couple to regret ever taking the initiative. I later learned that Rita, a fierce entrepreneur who would not sacrifice running her just budding private school might have backed down on her desire to birth the number of kids she and Luke had imagined. If handling only one child seemed like an uphill task, she said, they might as well forget about having one while focusing on Daniel.

The unsatisfied husband wouldn't have that and had left no stone unturned in looking for a quick-fix to their snowballing situation. A friend at work had directed them to my office to hear what I had to say about it before they jettisoned their familial goals.

Getting set to update the couple about the prevailing situation, I asked for the child's age. It turned out he was five and would turn six in the following month. I asked if they've heard of ADHD at any time, especially Rita who owned a school. She slurred. Amidst the constant distraction from the boy, I took both parents on a quick tour on behavioral disorders and how ADHD transpired.

They listened with keen interest as I drew out images of tables and charts highlighting the symptoms of ADHD. I have also presented relevant images in this chapter which describe the prevalent symptoms of ADHD in children. Table 1.0 & 2.0 display the changes in ADHD symptoms from childhood to adulthood.

Table 1.0[13]

1.	Preschool years	Primary	Adolescence	Adulthood
Inattention	• Short play • Sequences (<3 min) • Leaving activity incomplete • Not listening	• Brief activities (≤10 min) • Premature changes of activity • Forgetful; disorganized, distracted environment	• Less persistence than peers (<30 min) • Lack of focus on the details of a task • Poor planning ahead	• Details not completed • Appointments forgotten • Lack of foresight
Overactivity	"Whirlwind"	• Restless when calm expected	• Fidgety	• Subjective feelings of restlessness
Impulsivity	• Does not listen • No sense of danger (hard to distinguish from apposition ally)	• Acting out of turn; interrupting other children and blurting out answers • Thoughtless rule-breaking • Intrusions on peers; accidents	• Poor self-control • Reckless risk-taking	• Motor and other accidents • Premature and unwise decision-making • Impatience

Infancy/toddler years	<ul><li>Irritability, tendency to cry more than other children</li><li>Problems with sleep</li><li>Being 'fussy' with food</li><li>Restlessness</li></ul>
Pre-school/nursery years	<ul><li>Short attention span, for. ex. Struggling to listen to long stories</li><li>Mood swings, angry outbursts</li><li>Fine motor skill problems</li><li>Not interacting as much with other children</li></ul>
Primary School	<ul><li>Problems to sit quietly and follow rules</li><li>Problems with reading; struggling academically</li></ul>

	<ul><li>Problems collaborating with other children</li><li>Problems with concentration and focus</li></ul>
Secondary school	<ul><li>Ongoing problems with academic tasks</li><li>Tendency to challenge authority</li><li>Problems with time management</li><li>Forgetfulness</li><li>Being easily bored and distracted</li><li>Being impulsive and at times irritable</li><li>Engaging in risky behaviours (smoking, drinking, drugs, sexual experiences, etc)</li></ul>

Fig. 1.1

These behaviors interfere with a child's behavioral, social, cognitive, and emotional development. Thus, there's a need to spotlight them and understand how they handicap the child. Over the next few pages, I'll shine light on the major signs of ADHD in children from which you can draw insight on the best way to deal with it.

Inattentiveness

Tye's Mood

On one summer morning as I tidied my yoga patio, my phone buzzed. Not as expected. Just then it clicked that my mobile phone served as the alternative line since my office telephone had a broken conduit problem. My first inclination was to discard the call since it was only a few minutes past 7 am.

But on a whim, I got curious on why an unknown contact will decide to call before business time. The shaky voice cracked from the other side. It was a woman.

"Hey, Sharon. Do you think a child can be depressed…for how long???"

I thought to probe more on her identity but I stopped. Courtesy seemed immaterial at this moment. Her fluid voice cut deep into the layers of my heart and I knew I'd be sinning if I stopped her without hearing the entire conversation. I filled the silence with a fake cough and said,

"Well, it depends. What's the situation?"

For three days now, Tye, her seven-year-old girl had suddenly gone mute unwilling to talk to anybody or play or clean her room. The only time she voiced what sounded like words was to ask for a meal. And it turned out that she forgot the name of staple dishes whereas her parents depended on her ability to point out the food to know what she wanted.

"I understand," I said, "it's normal with kids going through a peculiar medical phase. I'd like to know: have you observed if she has behaved in a similar way before now?"

"Yes, she gets frequent Do-Not-Disturb days but it only lasts for a few hours. I began to notice this attitude in her after I finalized my divorce with my ex-husband. Must be her way of coping with the divorce, I thought. But it's been nearing three days now and my husband and I are out of our heads trying to figure out what could be wrong."

We met to further discuss that evening. I asked her to tell me of the other unusual signs she noted in her daughter. It happened that Tye had lost a precious star necklace that her paternal grandmother gave her during her last visit to her dad's. "While she was getting all worked up about it, I encouraged her to take it slow because she'd find it eventually. It's been almost five days now and the jewelry is not anywhere in sight. Then she slumped back into that DND dark hole."

I asked her to contact her ex-husband to see if Tye acted in the same way whenever she visited. She also filled the assessment form and got one for her dad too. After a close look at the submissions, it occurred to me that Tye could be suffering from ADHD disorders.

What to Look Out For

The symptoms of inattentive ADHD are easiest to miss or mistake as either a mental health condition or personality trait. Yet, this ignorance does little to bring out the truth and talk more of finding a solution. The National Institute of Mental Health posits that medical personnel often find it hard to recognize inattentive ADHD symptoms making it an underdiagnosed disorder whereby necessary treatment is scarce to children with the condition.

Children with this condition will demonstrate the following:

1. Careless Attention to Detail

Aside from the irrelevant, once-in-a-blue-moon, and easy-to-forget events that may punctuate each of our lives, children with inattentive ADHD fail to remember salient daily activities. For instance, they may forget to do tasks assigned to them or leave their homework in school causing the class teachers to blame them from time to time.

They have a working memory deficit which otherwise enables individuals to keep information for a long enough period of time until they use it. This deficit can lead to significant problems in daily activities. With this symptom in play, their daily routines often slip and may constantly require prompting to keep things in scope.

2. Difficulty in focusing

Hunger, stress, fatigue, or worry could lead to inability to focus one's attention. In the case of an ADHD child, all of these factors may or may not be in place to experience poor concentration. Speaking with mothers of ADHD children at a parenting workshop last year, one of the women reported that her eight-year-old lacked focus for boring activities like doing assignments but will hyper-focus in front of a video game he's interested in.

A way to rethink this difficulty is to view it as lack of control over what to focus on. The ADHD brain is always thinking about something and therefore struggles to stop at the instance of an "intrusion." Unless, of course, the intrusion is something they fancy which isn't often the case with the usual day-to-day activities.

Thus, there might be a need to reengineer the focus of the ADHD mind to what needs to be done now. Through this they can eradicate incomplete projects, zero-attention during conversations or zoning out in-between thoughts, and start practicing mindfulness and living a life that's full, rich, and rounded.

3. Disorganization

Organizing a task such as house chores or school work can seem overwhelmingly impossible for an ADHD child. Wherever there's a massive list of what to do, handle, or remember, the ADHD child can only escape this external chaos by causing an internal one that appears as mood swings, high stress levels, and anger. These silent struggles may give way to other people's judgments and blames.

At other times, the outcomes may be mild in the form of a messy room or locker, starting several creative projects while cluttering the elements out and about, or doing the laundry without folding it. Also, it shows up in constant forgetfulness, regularly misplacing things, or failure to follow instructions.

Many unsuspecting parents have categorized this latter behavior as that of a defiant child. But isn't this far from the case when talking about an ADHD child? A growing body of research is revealing that ADHD brains are unlike brains without ADHD. It states that the frontal cortex, basal ganglia, and parts of the cerebellum are usually smaller in ADHD brains than typical brains.

So, it makes sense that the next time your kid flaunts your orders, you want to be sure that it's not due to a medical condition they're battling with before dishing out rounds of punishments.

Hyperactivity

Mark's Impatience

Has your child got the firecrackers ever ready to launch it at anyone's face at any time? You're not alone. Mark's mom also thought her son was going nuts after he shut down his cousin's 15th birthday when they visited in the previous summer break.

Jaden's parents wanted to celebrate their daughter's fifteenth birthday in a grand style since it earmarked her departure into college.

Mark's mom thought Mark might like to see his cousin one last time before he heads to college himself. They had lived together in the neighborhood for years now and have been good friends with other children their age. They zoomed off in Simone's car after a quarrel over who gets to drive the new Hyundai Accent. Mark was a few months from sixteen but Simone wouldn't have him drive until he got his license.

A host of teenagers lurked around Jaden parent's yard in groups of three and four. Those who belonged in a larger group stood in pairs of two and busied themselves chatting away. Once Mark stepped out of the car, he hurried to meet a group of boys in such a frenzy that would have taken Simone aback if she were not used to her boy already. She clicked her tongue and shook her head as she double checked the car locks.

About twenty minutes into the party, an outburst broke out from the teen's camp. Simone would have sworn that it had something to do with Mark but prayed underneath her breath that not this time. Oops! Too late. In a flash, she saw Jaden had a scowl on her face as she captained half a dozen girls to the other end of the yard, away from Mark's rage.

It turned out that Mark sniffed a foul play from his bestie and girlfriend. He never waited to find out the truth before the ticking time bomb detonated. The mob tried to rescue the disoriented girlfriend from getting wound up in the fistful fight between the two teens. Maybe Jaden's party would have been salvaged if the crowd intervened earlier before someone got punched in the face and got his nose broken.

This last incident made Simone take the time to reflect on what kind of mother she had been raising Mark while his father served in the army. Would his husband be proud of the quick temper raving Mark's life aside from the fact that he suffered that too while they courted? Or was this a gene thing after all? On a quest to find out why Mark got sent home from play dates, had trouble sitting still, and found it excruciating waiting his turn; she turned to a child counselor who invited her to speak with me.

One microscopic look at Mark's life events exposed his condition in connection to ADHD. Simone realized she wasn't a bad mother after all and started to seek ways to help manage her child's tendencies. In the same way, for parent's dealing with 'Mark' whether at the infant, tween, or teenage stage; you may observe your child manifest the following behaviors:

1. Restlessness

If your child wouldn't stop running around, climbing things, or tripping over them or probably your teenager toughens it out with relaxing, it might just be another sign of ADHD. A child that rejects avenues to feel calm and catered for might just be manifesting restlessness that's an offshoot of hyperactivity.

Restless children would throw tantrums, hands, and fists to get what they want. And this isn't a case of eliminating discomfort by meeting their needs. Rather, it is the thrill of fighting to obtain their desires at every cost that characterize this behavior. They're ever on the go, way ahead of their turn, time, and energy.

It becomes obvious in frequent and excessive talking, inability to sit still, or trouble doing things quietly especially during downtimes. An ADHD child may pass on siesta or naps in favor of pressuring their peers to play with their toys.

2. Impulsivity

Interruptions and intrusion are the hallmark of an impulsive ADHD child. I like to view them as the unstoppable group of the ADHD disorders. There's little or no regard for situational social boundaries. Giving unsolicited opinions and inserting themselves into activities they were otherwise uninvited is norm with people with this type of ADHD.

The downside to this is they may fail to realize that people count this behavior as rude and unwanted. The ADHD child may be sorry and show deep apologies but that does little in taking away the urge to do so next time. It's inherent.

Completing a person's sentences before they have finished speaking, jumping into conversations before their turns, and other self-restraint problems might come off as irritating to others. Friends and classmates often deem it fit to count an ADHD kid out on social occasions.

Emotional irregularity

Few doctors will factor in emotional irregularity when diagnosing ADHD. The process of fasting on a feeling, insensitivity to others' emotions, oversensitivity to rejection and disapproval, bottling up fear, sadness and low self-esteem are all tied to ADHD.

Sometimes, an ADHD child wrestling with emotional irregularity can develop a gating mechanism for dealing with it whereby the child does not distinguish between dangerous threat and minor problem. Thus, even the nuanced things send the child to an automatic panic mode making the ADHD brains unable to deal with stressful and natural life events.

In explaining the whys and how ADHD stir up intense anger, feelings of frustration, and hurt, clinical psychologist at Yale, Thomas E. Brown puts a spin on it:

"Challenges with processing emotions start in the brain itself. Sometimes the working memory impairments of ADHD allow a momentary emotion to become too strong, flooding the brain with one intense emotion."

When you talk about ADHD, the truth is, emotions do rule. When Mark quarreled with his mom for disallowing him to drive her new car, when Tye got into the DND mode, and Daniel wouldn't listen to anyone—you could say they were all stuck in their emotions.

My grandson Mason always needs time out when things begin to seem out of hand and frustration starts to seep in. This overwhelming emotion could spring from refusal to join a rowdy grocery shopping or something along the lines. He ticks off with a yelp or cry and many a time, we let him cool off whenever he's caught in the bout of incessant and irritable cries. The result? A

Mason that's just a bit calm and ready to move on to the next activity.

You see, the working memory impairments of ADHD blows on a momentary emotion making it too strong, too intense compared to the situations that warranted it. On the flip side, this impairment rarely leaves the child with sufficient sensitivity toward the essence of expressing a certain kind of emotion since they have lost sight of the relevant information.

Is ADHD the same in all children?

Let's begin from the two major dichotomy—boys and girls. Boys exhibit external signs of hyperactivity that are typically considered the signs of ADHD. Girls are prone to be more withdrawn with self-esteem issues and as such, the signs are not overtly visible. Zeroing into how ADHD affects each individual child, we call on the awareness that ADHD is a neurodiverse disorder and so affects each person differently.

To best understand this uniqueness and impact of ADHD on each child, there is need to recognize the variability of each symptom which I'll discuss below.

Variability in ADHD symptoms

Various researchers have identified wide differences in ADHD characteristics that children display across various settings. Here's the truth: variability is outside of the child's control. Temporal situations and situational variables certainly influence the demonstrations of the symptoms in a child.

For instance, a momentary ADHD symptom in a child might not mean that the child has the disorder. In a real sense, it is the consistent display of the symptom overtime that becomes concrete evidence in labeling the ADHD child. Still in line, situations that elicit the same kind of ADHD behavior in a child every single time may offer insight about the ADHD stance of the child.

Indeed, the interplay of a consistent ADHD symptom in a given context overtime could bear witness that the child has ADHD.

Yet, the signs and symptoms observed within these contexts of time and setting can differ due to the following reasons:

1. Comorbid conditions

Just as no two neurodiverse brains are the same, you can say the same of the associated conditions that come with ADHD. I have earlier established in Chapter 1 that every ADHD case is accompanied with associated conditions called comorbid or co-existing conditions. Every child's comorbid condition is unique to them. And this constitutes the gaps and breaks that split the difference when dealing with diverse ADHD children.

a. Cognitive difficulties

Struggles in the mental faculty might hinder learning and is primarily due to conditions such as dyslexia, ODD, Tourrete, and its match, co-existing with ADHD in a child. This might result in problems with basic literary, speech, and language development, or time and spatial struggles if the child is dyslexic. Or it may affect the numerical skill, mathematical concepts, and mathematical sequences in any case of Dyscalculia in the child. Eventually, it leads the child to score lower than expected in class grades.

b. Affective difficulties

You'll agree that the mental state isn't the only affected region when we speak of neurodiversity. The behavior and emotion are also under the sphere of judgment. Bipolar disorder, depression, alcoholism, anxiety, and a horde of other behavioral disorders may travel in group with ADHD making the child have multiple comorbid diagnosis. Affective difficulties result in extreme self-esteem issues, emotional immaturity, and social skills problems.

2. Somatic situations

Many children with ADHD might be sensitive to touch, smell, noise, and a host of other stimuli. The variability in response depends on which one the child is most reactive to. The level of difficulty in dealing with cold, warmth, or sleep is also likely to determine how the child responds or reacts. I had a child in my office once that wouldn't stop smiling. He smiled when praised or scolded, awake or asleep. On the flip side, there are other kids who rarely smiled.

It is now clear that ADHD or any other kind of disorder affects different people differently.

What matters is to know and understand your ADHD child's unique disposition and be rest assured you can better address the challenges it poses as you seek to offer useful help.

Early signs and symptoms of ADHD can prove an overwhelming challenge. This chapter enlightened you on how ADHD is from your child's perspective. The next few pages will discuss your child's ADHD from your angle. You may find the next chapter speaking your mind from time to time: feel free to let the words leap into your heart regularly.

If you're feeling worn out, disoriented, and exhausted from parenting "a child that wouldn't listen," the truths saddled in the next chapter might make you sit at the edge of your seat as you find solace in the fact that you're not alone. And, of course, there might be a way around good parenting in the most unexpected scenarios after all.

KEY TAKEAWAY:

- ADHD behaviors interfere with a child's behavioral, social, cognitive, and emotional development.

- Children with inattentive ADHD will demonstrate careless attention to detail, difficulty in focusing, and disorganization

- Children with hyperactivity display restless and impulsive behaviors.

- Emotions do rule and oscillate within ADHD children

- No two ADHD children are the same. Each ADHD child has a unique comorbid condition(s) that differentiates their experience and behaviors.

CHAPTER THREE

COMMON CHALLENGES OF PARENTING AN ADHD CHILD

"Parenting has nothing to do with perfection. Perfection isn't even the goal, not for us, not for our children."- L. R. Knost

Chapter 2 connected you to an ADHD child on a deeper level. You familiarize yourself with the various outputs and manifestations that characterize a child with ADHD disorders. Through microscopic attention on how the signs of inattention, hyperactivity, and emotional irregularity show up to affect a kid, you found useful insight and information that justifies your child's ADHD behaviors.

Again, you discovered that no two ADHD kids are the same. And this reality owes to the factors that differ in the way they apply to children. Comorbidity conditions and somatic situations rank higher up the ladder of things that contribute to the differences and uniqueness of behavior from one child to another.

This Chapter will focus on the impact of parenting an ADHD child. I bet some pieces of this chapter might not meet you as a surprise. You may have to endure involuntary catharsis as you immerse yourself in the details of the story of parents broken down, torn apart, and bounded up again during their ADHD parenting journey.

If you've been anticipating the delicate layers of wounds and scars, scalds of frustration and furry, and stories of victory and triumph woven into my experience of raising a neurodiverse child and grandchild; then sit tight because it's high time you have it. I believe each one parent has a story to tell and anyone who has undergone an ADHD parenting might as well have a bit of silent history sitting in-between their ears.

I consider myself privileged to render such a story that resonates with thousands of parents out there and perhaps with you holding this book. Speaking your mind is of utmost delight and rare honor which I approach with sincere gratitude and sacred grace. You're about to flip through the pages of learning, unlearning, relearning, and eventual growth that took place in my life while I raced against the odds.

In my early days of dealing with an autistic kid, I longed for a book that discussed the negativity that trailed the paths of raising an ADHD child. I thought if I could just find one person who felt what I felt to give me a nudge or a word that would carry me through, that would make a huge difference. Well, I saw articles and literature that majored on ways to help ADHD children manage their behaviors. I encountered several thesis and research that bordered on signs and symptoms, treatments and theories, alongside multiple ways to handle the situation like a perfect parent.

No doubt they were pronounced in keeping me going. But I knew I needed something personal—I wanted that pat on the back from someone who has walked this path before. As I continued my fruitless search for empowerment and motivation, I encountered the breakthrough that flipped the switch.

I started journaling. Unlike the conventional way of keeping a journal, I think mine was out of style. My first journal was a rimmed A4 paperback. It was an honest mix of my soulful stories and key findings. I poured out my heart on the good and not-so-good days. I still found room to squeeze in my research in pieces and fragments. Somehow, they worked together and I may have immortalized this format as I still use it today.

These words you're about to read are excerpts from my journals. I hope you feel inspired, empowered, and energized as you digest the chunks of insights as I unveil them.

Dealing With Peter

After our first daughter's wedding celebration on one of the weekends that ended the summer in 2006, I stayed back to rest a while as I felt a heavy fatigue wrapping around me. My husband had beat the reception the previous day to meet up with an inevitable business meeting in San Antonio. So, I had to take the drive from Las Vegas to San Antonio, alone.

A few blocks away from our home, I pivoted into our family hospital for a check-up and get a few prescriptions. I couldn't express my shock when Gia suggested I took a pregnancy test. I giggled in embarrassment as if to say, "Watch it Gia, even if my first child is only twenty, she got wedded just yesterday and that's only saying I'm too old to birth a child by now."

Gia had worked in the hospital for a quarter century now and she must have read my expression. She flattened her thin Indian lips under her bright big eyeballs before she spoke. "Hey, Sharon…You're still looking as radiant as the first time I saw you twenty years back. Having a new member of the family isn't a bad idea. Go, I'll get you a nurse for your test immediately."

Positive. The pregnancy test was positive and I was three months gone. My children felt it was a good thing to have a new sibling. My husband did his best to calm my nerves regarding having another child after eight years since the last one. I thought it abnormal but he pressed further until I decided to see the brighter side.

Peter arrived in June. He was a stunning baby with vibrant energy. He cried hard, swung hard, and took no time in showing off infant strength and vigor. His eyes were alert and I felt he was a bit sensitive when breastfeeding except when in a quiet room. Everyone loved to pick him up but he loved crying much more.

His cries soon turned into unruliness as he grew into a toddler. He took him time before he responded to people calling him "Peter." He kicked against simple orders and continued playing in a particular kind of way with his toys. He often busied himself with banging the throw pillows and showed indifference when his throws hit. I never counted that as anything but just a child's play.

Months passed and by the time he was fifteen months, he didn't smile when you looked at him and didn't talk much. I tried to suppress the only meaning that crept into my mind because of this behavior: that I had a son that was a broken and spoiled child. I swallowed hard. What? How did I raise a rebel? But I kept mute about it trying to find ways to call my boy to order.

By the time I enrolled Peter into Kindergarten when he was 3 years old, his teacher complained about him not picking up on language like the others. She had taught my older children and never for once nurtured such a comment. I had no idea what to make of the situation but resolved to put in more effort regarding his homework.

The more I tried to make him responsive to learning, the harder the toll on me with no tangible results to show. Although he seemed to enjoy the entire process of repetition or recitation, he lacked the power to remain on cue when interrupted or whenever he retired from that activity.

Going the hard way, I threatened to take away a cookie if he mixed up his alphabets, yet I couldn't trace any fear in his eyes. He slept on a whim and comfortably ate late in the night. I thought his behavior was rude and uncalled for. And the complaints? They kept coming in spades. My husband and two sons thought he'd catch up even but I had a different opinion.

So, I rolled back my sleeves and began the dirty work. I searched the internet to get an answer for my baby's state. None of my children had displayed such a lackadaisical attitude as a child or teen and Peter wouldn't be different. On my first day of conducting my research, I hit upon an idea that left me with mixed feelings.

It was a statistic that showed the frequency at which parents reported that their child had ASD. The figure showed an increase from about 5.5 to 11.6 per 1000 children. I further drilled into the characteristics of ASD and you can guess it: it fit into Peter's disposition. Initially, I felt clueless on what to do with the information. I decided to research deeper and longer for stretches of time.

Like an escaping steam, I breathed when I discovered that I may not have been responsible for Peter's disruptive behavior. And in fact, beating myself or Peter up wasn't the exact solution I needed. A gust of motherly empathy swept through me as I browsed for ways to administer all the help he needed.

Soon, I brought my family up to speed on the current situation and kept abreast with my research. Interacting with consultants, practicing what I learned, contacting other parents with neurodiverse children became my new routine. I got lost immersed in the process of finding the best aid for my child and I'm super glad today that I took the chance.

Disruptive Behavior, Attention Deficit, Impulsivity

Christine's third child Mason came in 2017. Not too long after his birth, Christine fell into an episode of worry that I could recognize at once. She would call me over the phone to describe how she's having a hard time getting along with her child. Mason kicked hard, cried hard, and slept the lightest. He blabbered incessantly and wouldn't sit still anywhere else but the rocking chair. I knew those signs.

Recently when Mason was in a school going age last year, I began my research with his class teacher. Mason did well in his class works and home works. The only thing his teacher pointed out was his inability to focus every time. Mason would either play with toys, chatter, or trouble other kids.

I think my line of consulting with parents of neurodiverse children took flight with my own child—Christine. Sometimes, when she called to talk about the void and powerlessness she felt whenever Mason defied her orders in the presence of grown-ups or other kids, I opened up to her in the same words that I will now uncover to you.

Here's the kicker: parenting an ADHD child could make you feel ripped off from any control you have over your child. This feeling is valid since just like your child, you have zero control over ADHD behaviors. Where does it get tricky? Most parents relinquish all influence due to frequent disobedience of the child. But there are some places where you do have control outside of the core ADHD behaviors.

The point where you can get involved is just beyond the core ADHD circle. Talk about helping your child manage ADHD at home, school, or extra-curricular activities, this is where your ability to control shines the most. You may consider letting go of any strategy that coerces change and execute those that promote correction where possible.

Academic Problems

Parents possess natural empathy toward their children which creates the desire to ease pains and give urgent solutions. Michelle's 12-year-old stepson, Chase, got diagnosed with ADHD in kindergarten. As a little boy, Chase was out of control and never followed authorities. He lacked coordination and always forgot about his homework. Most of all, he got into trouble in class and hit other children at will until his eventual suspension.

Michelle narrated how her heart sank when she learned about Chase's suspension. Although she had often gotten into fights with Chase regarding bathing, doing his homework, helping out with chores, she had taken Chase as a child and wondered if there was a remedy to Chase's disobedience.

Prior to the time, Michelle and her husband had no idea of ADHD. But Chase soon got diagnosed with the disorders and a lot of unsaid questions became answered. His relationship with Michelle transported from being a tug of war to a harmonious rhythm of calm, peace, and understanding. Since that time forward, Chase's memories stayed refreshed concerning the things that mattered and needed to be done. For instance, Michelle wrote on a dry-erase board to remind him of what's next on the agenda. It looked something like this: "time to take a bath, time for homework…"

Chase's parents developed a routine plan tailored to suit his conditions as an ADHD and ODD child. They never allowed him to jump into his homework right off after school. Instead, they differed this period giving him ample time to reboot and also introduced breaks that enabled him to work for ten minutes and steer clear for a few. The parents ultimately managed Chase's ADHD condition when they agreed to integrate available treatment.

Organizational Difficulties

It is true that our habits define who we are. While many parents of ADHD children tend to ask, "What's wrong with my child?" Carl's shocking question was: "What's wrong with me?" Before you begin with your own line up of questions, let's take a look at the backdrop of Carl's story.

Carl, 39, and father to his only 6-year-old child, Jeremiah, recently diagnosed with ADHD in the same year his mother was deployed to give health care during the COVID-19 pandemic. Mi as he's often called required an intensive approach of routines to steady his day-to-day activities. The moment he opened his eyes at dawn to when he rested them at dusk, he only operated within a regimented environment. Carl had heard his wife mention for the umpteenth time over the phone that those scheduled activities needed to be in place for their son to live a successful life. Believing that he had to put up with this for the rest of his life, childhood was the hardest part. He never thought he was made to last.

Two years down the lane, the work-from-home dad had become Jeremiah's best pal. Carl had internalized the flow of Mi's activities, immersed himself in its demands, and knew the tenets of the schedules even better than Mi's mom. Everything went on smoothly in a wave of unbroken commitment and elastic adjustments wherever it might be needed. Then Easter 2022 brought a realization that seemed far out of the blue.

On Easter Friday, Carl received an invitation from an old friend and colleague who just moved downtown. His wife and child had gone to celebrate with their family out of town and he had some leisure time away from work, so he accepted. Collin first noticed Carl's weird behavior on Easter's eve morning when Carl rolled out of the bed with no particular occupation even after being awake since two hours earlier.

Night came with an overwhelming activeness that prevented Carl from settling into sleep. It seemed like Carl's internal body clock was out of sync with the standard sleeping and waking time. Collin couldn't help but bring up the discussion on Easter Sunday over a home-made glazed ham and jamin cipollinis. "You weren't like this when last we pulled an all-nighter before the COVID in my former apartment."

It hit Carl that keeping up with Mi's schedules and appointments for managing his disorganization might have as well rubbed off on him. Now he would have to live like that for probably another stretch of years until their child matures. But did he mind?

Self-esteem Troubles and Social skills Deficits

Olivia had a class presentation by mid-term. Her teacher had her parents mailed together with other classmates' parents.' Right from age 5, Olivia had been diagnosed with inattentive ADHD and mostly found herself less and less attracted to public speaking on many fronts. Olivia's parents had informed her school of her diagnosis and the school had risen to the occasion of helping out with a progressive learning environment and a supportive class.

When she learned of the compulsory class presentation, she felt her tommy tie in a knot. The highest she had gone with public speaking was answering a question in class while teachers and classmates applauded. At home, Olivia's parents told her incredible things and let her know that even if she would fall silent anytime she had to be on stage, they would remain her greatest cheerleader.

Olivia's parents often caught her in an anxious state where she shivered in her pants if stressed, afraid, or panicky. They worried that Olivia would be unable to participate in the class presentation and may have to go with a substitute test. Beyond their biggest fears, Olivia walked in on her parents two weeks before mid-term to declare her intents of speaking during the class presentation.

The wheels dug in in rotation. Intense preparation took the stage and Olivia practiced her speech for a thousand times over before the D-Day. All these, she did side by side while administering her medication. Her parents reached out to Olivia's ADHD consultant on how best to maximize this special period of her life. The consultant never thought twice before she walked them through the process with much patience.

On the big day, Olivia's parents asked if they could come and although it was an all-pupil's activity, her teacher made an exception. Olivia was the first to present. She may have skipped a few lines and mixed-up words, but she exceeded the expectations of her audience who knew about her history.

Certainly, Olivia's parents may not be present during her interpersonal conversations. Yet, they have succeeded in raising a kid that dared to vie for a reality far out of her current circumstance.

There are a few, if not *0. percentage* of children with ADHD today that can replicate Olivia's daring behavior. The logic behind her action could be attributed to the fact that most of her ADHD symptoms are not overly active or impulsive like that of her hyperactive male counterpart. While this might not be scientifically proven, it well represents a real experience in the grand scheme of ADHD.

As I wrap up, I hope this chapter has, first of all, made you recognize that you're not alone in your journey. I am convinced that more than ever before, you have seen through the lenses of these stories and etched out a favorable personality with which to handle ADHD events with your child.

Chapter 4 will underscore ideas about how to incorporate learning that suits your child's condition.

KEY TAKEAWAY:

- Just like your child, you have zero control over ADHD behaviors. Yet, you don't have to relinquish your power because you feel powerless. Instead, drive every ounce of control toward helping your child.

- Early diagnosis and finding immediate help for your child can foster real parent-child bond.

- Taking care of your ADHD kid may leave indelible imprint in your habits and schedules. Accept your child and embrace the challenge that accompanies carrying for them.

- Positive words and powerful beliefs in your child can strengthen their mindset and give them wings to fly.

CHAPTER FOUR

HELPING YOUR CHILD MANAGE ADHD

"The very traits that once held Ty back are now his greatest assets."

Yvonne Pennington, mother of Ty Pennington

In the previous Chapter, I reviewed stories of parents' struggles and challenges in dealing with an ADHD child. I bet that many of the testimonials in the past chapter ring true with you too. You saw the influence and impact of the disorder beyond the scope of the child to how it affects the parents.

A vital idea expressed was that ADHD is difficult for either the child or parent to control. Yet, there's how parental help comes in handy—that is, the sphere of influence that an ADHD child parent can manage the child's disorders.

Remember Michelle and Chase from Chapter 3? Michelle and her husband chose to medicate Chase which led to a massive improvement in Chase's condition. Michelle narrated how they battled the thought of putting little Chase on medication in kindergarten. When they eventually went for it, Michelle reported that to see Chase medicated and non-medicated was "two different children."

According to Michelle, "You can tell the minute it kicks in: He goes from bouncing up and down and not following directions—he can't even complete simple tasks without prompting—to being focused and calm. He can process thoughts; he can do his homework. It's a whole different world."

There's a right way to take charge of your circle of influence and act in a way that improves and corrects your child's condition and below are a handful of proven strategies.

Level 1 - Strategies to Help Your Child Become Focused

The primary shortcoming of most ADHD children is the inability to focus. And just as I discussed in Chapter 2, we discover that the ADHD child focuses on the wrong and unimportant things.

Your duty is to recalibrate their focus on things that are important and serve them.

Many issues like hyperactivity, forgetfulness and the like crowd under the umbrella of conditions that can be readily treated by a focus reordering. Consider implementing the following strategies to redirect your child's focus.

1. Make a to-do list

One of the commonest habits you'll find among ADHD children is routine keeping. It's time to transform this strength into a working process to help curb lack of focus. Stories of ADHD parenting attest to the fact that introducing and committing to a regimented style helps their child to cope and get through each day while doing the right things at the right time.

In case you don't fancy Michelle's method of instruction via easy-dry board, you might find a few apps super cool like Joon, Homey, Cozi, Our Home, Chore Pad, and Todoist.

2. Try memory exercise games

Games are engaging on many levels whether intellectual, physical, or psychological. They act as fun ways to boost your child's cognitive skill. Some games that the entire family can try include:

- Word recall: say a series of words and have your child immediately repeat them after you. Ask questions about the order of words and see if they can catch up or not.

- Card match: This concentration game involves matching pairs of cards. Make sure your child can access these cards to begin pairing them.

- Picturizing: Have a pool of pictures arranged and organized in a linear line. Ask your child to study the progression of these pictures. Tell them to imagine the images in their mind. You can go a step further by shuffling the pictures and asking them to guess which ones fell out of place.

3. Stack and break down

It's seamless to flow in-between similar tasks rather than jump across unrelated ones. Identify similar tasks in your child's life and group them together as you encourage them to do each task one at a time.

A 2019 study notes that the human brain is incapable of multitasking and works more efficiently when tasks are approached one by one. Stacking tasks and breaking them down into bits and pieces naturally matches the tempo and rhythm of an ADHD child.

4. Coffee in small doses

Repantis, Bovi, Ohla, Kuhn and Dresler revealed in their 2021 study that coffee can positively enhance and sustain attention, provided it is taken moderately. High consumption leads to anxiety, nervousness, and inability to stay focused.

5. Lockdown social media

For children old enough to operate their mobile phones, you want to make sure that reboot breaks in-between tasks are not squandered on social media. What you want to do is to eliminate distractions which can constantly pop up when using social media.

Level 2- Strategies to Keep Your Child Motivated

You've heard about how your ADHD child's emotion can be a stronghold or weak link in their day-to-day activities. Positive emotions source and reinforce motivations that help to keep children going.

1. Give praise for effort made

You want your child to take control of their task, right? Then praise your child using a format that elevates effort over ability and watch your child soar and improve. Praising your child for completing a task rather than rewarding them for the results obtained will go a long way in sustaining interest in doing the task and staying consistent.

2. Make your child the decision-maker

No one enjoys being tossed around. Nobody likes to be nagged to perform a chore or task. Give your child enough freedom to decide when to start a task, how long they think it will take, and have them compare the reality and their prediction in the end. Notice how this encourages your child to start and finish major tasks.

3. Set goals

Setting goals has never harmed anyone but to help. Create a vision board unique to your child. Let their personality come alive and make it fun. They could hang cut out pictures or printed web images of where they want to go and what they want to achieve at the end of the school week, term, and year.

4. Connect bland events to interesting ones

We all have our fun things to do and so do ADHD children! A father accompanied an ADHD child to a camp meeting in hopes of bonding together. For the life of the father, his son was rather interested in unthinkable things like anthills and daffodils and butterflies, spending most of his time observing and admiring.

Nothing changed until the father decided to connect to the boy on his own level. He took interest in his child's hobbies and that broke the ice. Recognize what your child loves—might be baseball or video games or cooking—and relate the uninteresting events like learning mathematics or literature to it.

5. Give movement allowance

Sitting still over quiet tasks bores an active mind. Make room for stand breaks, walk breaks, or talk breaks when your child is engaged in a monotonous task. It might look something like infusing a "music-time" midway in completing a math assignment.

As an additive, I have provided a list of ten things to never say to your ADHD child as suggested by ADHD experts at ADDitude

1. You're Stupid…

2. I Love You, But…

3. Why Can't You Be Normal?

4. If Only You'd Apply Yourself…

5. Clearly, You Didn't Take Your Meds Today

6. I Wouldn't Wish An ADHD Child on Anyone

7. You Should Be Ashamed

8. You're Just Like Your Father

9. (Sarcastic Remarks at Irrational Behaviors)

10. I Hate You

Level 3: Strategies To Keep Your Child Educated

Helping others in key positions understand your child's condition and needs is a profound step in ensuring your child receives great education. Teachers, guardians, and coaches are inevitable caregivers that can help your child make judicious use of their education and other learning opportunities. Consider the following steps in achieving quality education for your ADHD child.

1. Talk to your child's teachers

Letting in your child's teacher on your child's ADHD condition is no rocket science. Just go by the rules that are considered normal and acceptable within your social context.

- Never shame or blame the teacher for not picking the cues or not trying their best to make your child better. Rather, enlighten them on the social and emotional effect of ADHD and how it can cause challenges in learning, motivation, and behavior.

- Lend a helping hand as the job of educating your ADHD child doesn't lie exclusively with the teacher. Be open to answer teachers' questions and provide adequate resources that might help to better understand your child's needs.

- You might need to get a form that puts explanations in concise and concrete writing. The teacher can refer to this in your absence.

2. Explore Individualized Education Plus (IEP)

Care for a simple and short definition? An IEP helps children with specific disabilities like ADHD receive personalized educational assistance. The moment a child gets referred for this special assistance, a written plan is drawn and shared among a team of teachers, parents, and guardians.

Usually, the IEP evaluation process kicks off as soon as a caregiver recognizes that a child struggles in school. Then the IEP services such as auditory services, occupational therapy, parent counseling training, psychological services, children recreation, and school health services are employed to draft a unique plan that offers accommodation to ADHD children in a classroom setting.

Every neurodiverse child needs to get a form of extra support termed accommodation that's catered for within the IEP. Sitting accommodations, instructional accommodations, test-taking accommodations, and assignment accommodations are all vital artilleries in the IEP arsenal targeted toward a rich and considerate education system for your child.

The forward Chapter projects a framework for dealing with ADHD stigma. The suggestions and deliberations outlined will arm you with the right knowledge to help set the pace for your child's happiness in a critical world.

KEY TAKEAWAY:

- The quality of help a child receives equals the quality of life enjoyed. Setting up a to-do list, trying out memory games, breaking down tasks, regulating diets, and locking down social media are invaluable ways to help your child stay focused.

- Keep your child motivated by giving praise, granting ownership, setting goals, sustaining interests, and encouraging movement.

- Access special education needs for your child by exploring the necessary opportunities.

CHAPTER FIVE

SETTING THE PACE FOR YOUR CHILD'S HAPPINESS

"No medicine cures what happiness cannot"- Gabriel Garcia Marquez

By walking you through a three-level strategy, I helped you understand how you can help your child manage ADHD. Enforcing the Level-1 strategy for helping your child focus, applying the Level-2 strategies to keep your child motivated, and implementing the Level-3 strategies to assist your child in gaining a personalized education will lead to a life of fulfillment and order for your child.

This Chapter is designed to deliver the details you need to deal with ADHD stigma in yours or your child's life. More than that, you will find a working framework on the methods you can rely on to nurture and reinforce your child's social skills.

Nobody knew the pain of a disability nor the sting of its stigma as much as Mateo did. 32-year-old with a job as a Fashion Stylist in the luxury industry. He walks home with a heavy paycheck of $60,000 a month and knew he was worth every dollar because boy was, he good at his job! On diverse occasions, he got gigs to work with top brands and the gigs kept coming.

Loved and admired by all and sundry, there was no space reserved in Mat's life for an enemy, well, except himself. For although Mat seemed to have attained the pinnacle of his career, he lacked one crucial skill that would cost him the fortune of a lifetime!

Mat's company had sat as the industry champion when it came to fashion and styling. It's other branches of brand ambassador, brand strategist, brand manager, e-commerce manager have been doing well to climb to the top of the ladder, but not very much like the fashion category. In most cases, the celebratory awards the company raked in came on the wings of the styling and fashion department; thanks to the brilliant works of their all-time star, Mateo.

Mateo was the company's gem and excellent to a fault. The one clog in Mat's wheel, however, was his epileptic late coming: to meetings, to client's big day? He did that well. But what he was also good at his job and the myriad of awards tied to his name intensely made up for his weakness. The truth was, Mat wished on many occasions that he could stop showing up late. But he couldn't help it. The feeling of staying in bed for the next three hours after his alarm went off was bliss. And in Mat's eyes, nothing could compare to that!

Of course, he was used to the witty phrase of early to bed and early to rise right from his childhood. Even if he didn't want to hear about it, his mother wouldn't let him. Yet was it even his fault? He never neared sleep on any night until it was well past midnight. So, it followed that he woke up late, every morning for how many years now? 30? 32? Whatever age it was when he began to be conscious of himself—he had slept late and woke up late up to date.

Funny thing is, the ton of advice Mat had received about how lateness could lead to failure never bothered him. For what's the worry if they never worked on him? Now, the most sought-after fashion stylist in America, flying across the world to deliver his skill set to hungry clients, and currently the topmost breed in his industry; he had absolutely nothing to fear. This year's final gig was about creating a space and cementing him at the helm of affairs in his company and he looked forward to it.

On this year's final trip to style a French influencer, he let his guard down. A few days to Christmas, Mat woke up on that chilly Tuesday morning tucked in flannel sheets in the extravagant hotel room he had lodged. The clock struck 4 and he stopped the alarm. The very act initiated him into his dreamy hours where he did nothing but to turn and toss and let his mind wander.

The next time he looked, 12 past eight. What in the world was he thinking about that he lost track of time?!!!! He bounced out of bed and fell back right in his leg and he lost his balance. Not today, he whined. Would he have realized he was sick if he had obeyed that noisy alarm for once? He imagined all the faces eagerly waiting for his arrival by now. The buyouts client, the composite card photographer, the fashion model…The list was endless "They'll all just go on and wait as usual. Mat will be ready for them in the nick of time." He beamed.

Mat made his VIP entrance into the hollow skyscraper and gunned for the changing room at once. As he approached, he thought every glance carried layers of shady meaning beneath it and he wouldn't know why until he flunked into the dress room and saw his personal assistant sizing up, matching and pairing outfits. He had been replaced.

His legs felt like noodles and he couldn't stand it anymore. Mat hit the floor and, in a few minutes, landed in the hospital. From that time forward, he never ran out of erratic behaviors, blackmailing anyone the company sent to replace him at any gig event. The once *dearest* Mat was fast transitioning into Mat the *dreaded*. On one of his frequent visits to the hospital, he got into an impatient conversation with a consultant letting him know of his desire for a quick fix to his unrestrained impulses. It was at this point that Mateo discovered he has ADHD.

News flew around and his company got a whiff of it. On the platform that ADHD had no cure and the risk that Mat might continue pulling new stunts due to his 'illness,' they decided to let him go. Mat collapsed when he heard of his relief. His entire career sunk in his face and he couldn't bear watching it crumble. Clearing his desk turned out to be the most delusional day of his life. Everywhere he looked, people—his colleagues, juniors, and seniors—seemed to have something to whisper about. Was it his ADHD or his job termination? Where were his friends? Was the world waiting for this dark moment? He would never know. The once prosperous and energetic Mat, now tired and torn, retired at 32 to live a silent life while managing his fate and his fears.

Dealing with ADHD stigma

Up to eight kinds of stigma can be identified in our world: self-stigma, public stigma, perceived stigma, structural stigma, health practitioner stigma, label avoidance, associative or affiliate stigma. Each named stigma can show up in the case of ADHD.

Self-stigma may occur in children when they try to correct an embarrassing ADHD tendency without success. The stigma shifts to the public when society displays overarching sentiments about ADHD. Perceived stigma happens when you think people around will negatively judge you for having a particular trait. You're being structurally stigmatized when an institution deals with you based on policies founded on stigmatizing attitudes.

Health practitioner stigma plays out when a professional's belief about race, gender, or other stereotypes hinders him from giving effective care. Label avoidance occurs when a person or people distance themselves from a stigmatized group. Associative stigma aims at the people connected to a stigmatized group.

ADHD stigma materializes in the myths and bigotries that society wrongly believes about ADHD. For instance, saying ADHD is as a result of bad parenting or that people with ADHD are overmedicated. From the discussion in Chapter 1, it is evident that these myths are untrue and lacking facts.

To be free from the hold of ADHD stigma, sensitize your child on what is true concerning ADHD. Debunk the myths and guide them to the factual elements that support the validity of their condition.

Teaching & Reinforcing Social skills

This might be a cliché but it is ever so true: human beings are social animals. Even the most inattentive ADHD child ever requires a moderate use of talk to carry on and feel alive. Come to think of it, many of the ADHD child peers who stigmatize them do so for a primary reason.

It is because the ADHD child lacks the needed skill to communicate "normally" like everyone else. The following tips will help to scale your child's social skills.

1. **Develop listening skills**

Every typical individual I know loves to talk about themselves whether in therapy or out of it. And it is fascinating to know that majority of the people talked but have not learned to listen. Finding someone who genuinely listens in a fast-paced, quick-fix, digital world is hard to come by. Listening is the virtue that allows others to feel comfortable sharing their ideas and inputs.

Teach your child to become a good listener by maintaining regular eye contact, using non-verbal communication, and asking questions.

2. Practice empathy

Empathy isn't a strong suit for an ADHD child. As you have discovered earlier in this book in the section that dwelt on emotional irregularity, it's either a sharp spike in the intensity of emotion or a sheer low. There is hardly ever a moderation unless through an external influence of medication.

The first step toward learning to empathize is paying attention. Solving the attention puzzle puts the other party and the subject of discussion in focus in a way that your child can feel what others are saying and not just hear.

3. Engage with others

All of life is reciprocal. Give someone and they'll return the good will. In the same vein, speaking to someone means being spoken to.

Learn to engage your child in conversations by asking them questions and ask them to do the same to their classmates and friends. It's not going to be easy but by taking baby steps and embracing the challenge that novelty brings, they are liable to master the art overtime.

Studies credit low self-esteem, inability to succeed at a young age, and trouble making friends as an offshoot of untreated and unmanaged ADHD. Also, just as we have observed in the case of Mateo, ADHD can go on to produce relationship, work, and general life strain if left unchecked and untreated.

Does your child need medication or therapy? Or should that totally be out of your options? The next chapter answers these questions and similar ones. It proposes medical as well as non-pharmacological alternatives to help treat your child's ADHD.

KEY TAKEAWAY:

- Ignorance of ADHD conditions is a setback for ADHD children. Parents who diagnose their children early and sensitize them on the same pave the way for a great esteem in their child.

- The feelings of hurt, pain, and frustration common with stigma can only fester in your child's eyes if you fail to orientate them about their condition.

- Everyone can stigmatize your child but make sure it's not you.

- Recalibrate and improve your child's social skills by teaching them to listen, practice empathy, and engage with others.

CHAPTER SIX

THERAPY AND MEDICATION

"Wherever the art of medicine is loved, there is also love of humanity." - Hippocrates

ADHD can pose a threat to a child's life on countless occasions especially if undiagnosed early in life; if brutally stigmatized in a child, and if it's untreated. The early chapters of this book granted insights on how to spot ADHD in a child. The past chapter unveiled the dangers of stigmatization and how to live above it. This chapter closes in on the final reason—treatment.

Managing ADHD doesn't end with the parents. It is instead a coordinated efforts of a team of healthcare professionals, specialists, doctors, educators, and parents. It's important for you to help your child follow primary and practical ways to manage their ADHD. What's equally important is to rally support from educators, medical professionals, and mental practitioners to ensure optimum development for your child.

The Reward of Therapy

I like to view therapy as extended parenting. Do you think you've given your child a solid groundwork to help control behavioral lapses? Odds are you may be lagging behind on other fronts. How do you transform your child's negative emotions and thought patterns to positive ones?

Do you feel an overwhelming sense of helplessness and worry excessively as you parent your ADHD child? Chances are right now; you need a shoulder to lean on and a hand to walk you through the uncertain and trying times. Records show that mental health therapy is useful for about 75% of people who find it.

Regardless of the many misconceptions about therapy, the rewards are enormous! A great therapy session will provide you with any of these:

- A better understanding of your mental health

- Recognizing triggers of unhealthy behaviors

- Cultivating and improving interpersonal relationships

- Overcoming fears and coping with stress

- Creating a personal plan for mental health crisis and developing wellness goals

- Creating routine and stability

Finding The Right Therapist

The American Psychological Association (APA) estimates about 85,000 licensed psychologists in the US. To find one that's just right for you, you need to engage in a search by

- Asking trusted family and friends

- Asking your primary healthcare givers or contacting your community mental health center

- Searching online for psychologists or therapist's websites

- Using a trusted online directory such as APA's Psychologist Locator Service

In selecting from the pool of therapists, you want to consider one that aligns with your budget, yours and your child's schedules and also your personal preferences.

Closely related to booking a therapy appointment is joining a support group. Plenty support groups are functional either online or onsite and some operate both. Find out the ones that best fulfills yours or your child's community needs and get ready for a warm welcome.

Medications for ADHD

ADHD medications can be split into pharmacological and non-pharmacological treatments. The former is divided into two categories namely stimulants and non-stimulants. Psychostimulants—methylphenidate and amphetamines—are the most studied drugs for ADHD.

Similarly, there are two classes of non-stimulant drugs used in ADHD—the noradrenaline reuptake inhibitor atomoxetine and the a2-adrenergic agonists clonidine and guanfacine. FIG 6.1 and 6.2 below describe stimulant and non-stimulant medication respectively.

Drug	Duration type	Brand name *	Dosage schedule	Approximate duration of action (hours)	Typical starting dose	Maximum daily dose
	Short-acting	Ritalin, Metadate, Methylin	BID to TID	3-5	5	60
		Focalin	BID-TID	2-3	2.5	20
	Intermediate acting	Rital SR, Metadate ER, Methylun ER	QD to BID	3-8	10	60

	Extended release	Metadate CD, Ritalin LA	QD	6-8	10	60
		Concerta	QD	8-12	18	72
		Focalin SR	QD	12	5	30
		Daytrana	Patch worn for up to 9 hours		10	30
Amphetamines	Short-acting	Dexedrine spansule	BID to TID	4-6	5	30
		Adderall	QD to BID	4-6	5	40
	Intermediate-acting	Dexedrine spandsule	QD to BID	10	5	40
	Extended release	Adderal-XR	QD	10	10	30

		Vyva nse	QD	13	30	70

Key: QD: once a day; BID: twice a day; TID: three times a day

All may not be available in some countries and brand names may be different

FIG 6.1

Drug	Duration type	Brand name*	Dosage schedule	Typical starting dose (mg)	Maximum daily dose (mg)
Guanfacine	Extended release	Intuniv	QD	1	Age 8-12: 4 13-17: 7
Clonidine	Extended release	Kapway Catapres	BID	0.1	0.4 split in two doses
Atomocetine	Short acting	Strattera	QD to BID	70 kg or less: 0.5 mg/kg	70 kg or less: 1.4 mg/kg or 100

				Over 70 kg: 40 mg	Over 70 kg: 100 mg
Key: QD: once a day; BID: twice a day; TID: three times a day All may not be available in some countries and brand names may be different					

FIG 6.2

The second kind of medication that works well for your child is the non-pharmacological medication. This can be an alternative or addition to medications in cases where children do not respond to medication, are too young to take medication or lack access to it. It can also come in handy when you are keen to address certain comorbidity issues or medication that have significant adverse effect.

In such situations, options that can be explored include: behavioral and psychological treatment, neurofeedback, computerized cognitive training, dietary intervention and brain stimulation.

How do I know if my child needs medication?

The aim of any medication is to give children a chance at the best outcomes in life regardless of their limitations or delimitations. If you think that your child's symptoms haven't improved with counseling or behavior therapies alone, then your next go-to might be pharmacological medication.

Your child's age can be a factor to consider when deciding whether or not to medicate your child. Children under 6 years old can do well with non-pharmacological medications. However, between 70-80% of ADHD children show fewer symptoms when taking the fast-acting medications which are mostly stimulants.

When medication fails: side-effects

Can science fail? Maybe. Every medication has its side effects and that of ADHD isn't an exception. The commonest kinds of adverse effects of stimulants are mild, dependent, and transitory in the forms of insomnia, headaches, irritability, agitation, nervousness, tremor, loss of appetite, nausea, and weight loss. In order to combat these adverse effects, regulating doses or changing stimulant drugs could help.

In severe cases, sudden death and growth retardation is the end result. Stimulants have been studied to be prone to retard children's growth and reduce final adult height. Parents and drug administrators should be on the same page when discussing hot button issues as this. The remedy for growth retardation might be to take a break from medication during summer break as children resume growth when they stop stimulant intake.

It is necessary to ascertain risk factors when determining the kinds of drugs and medication to place a child on. While there is no known evidence that usage of ADHD drugs can increase the risk of cardiovascular attacks, a child's heart rate and blood pressure should be closely monitored at specific periods. That is, the beginning of the medication usage, after each dose change, and after every six months.

Any history of cardiac risk factors in the family should attract the prescription of a non-stimulant as an alternative. And on extreme occasions, parents should avoid medication and stick to the traditional methods for coping with ADHD. The table by Fewell. & Deutscher summarizes ways to cope with ADHD both at home and in school.

- View the child as a good child with a special need

- Remember that the child's misbehavior is organic in nature

- Capitalize on the child's strengths and emphasize the positive

- Provide a special time for the child each day

- Plan ahead when introducing new concepts and for challenging situations

- Reduce environmental distractions and be an alert listener

- Establish clear rules and apply them consistently

- Ensure that adults support the rules

- Secure eye-contact before giving directions

- Give clear, simple, straightforward directions

- Check child's understanding of directions and the consequences of failing to follow them

- Be patient and low key but firm

- Act, don't over talk

- Refrain from being drawn into debate or argument

- Use good and consistent behavior management techniques

- Understand and use time outs if the results are effective

- Give positive feedback and praise frequently and quickly after appropriate behavior

- Help the child recognize his or her own strength and accomplishments.

KEY TAKEAWAY:

- ADHD cure is not compulsory but treatment is necessary.

- Staying emotionally fit is good for your child's wellbeing as well as yours. Be open to using a therapy and social support as you deem fit.

- Go for medication if counsel and support fail.

CONCLUSION

Books are great ways to acquaint yourself with unfamiliar subjects. Certainly, the pages of this book have transported you from the uninformed valley of guess-work and assumptions about ADHD to the heights of factual and proven insights, saddled on the helms of first-hand experience. The above pages have demystified ADHD and dissolved every doubt you may have before picking up this book.

Much more, the various chapters served to consolidate prior knowledge that resonates with the truth. And it equally identifies and discards lies that could serve as barriers to parenting your ADHD child in the most loving and considerate ways.

In Chapter 1, you learned about what ADHD really is and gained expert knowledge on its background and how it works. This chapter explored information about the types and causes of ADHD, provided in-depth knowledge on who diagnoses ADHD, when, and how, and boldly debunk several myths about ADHD.

Chapter 2 discussed the various symptoms that appear in ADHD children as they transition into adulthood. You found out how these symptoms play out in your child's life and ways they may hinder daily activities. Through the lenses of other children's stories, you understood the diverse outlets that ADHD could manifest. Furthermore, the chapter closes with the mindset that each ADHD child is unique in the ways they display their behaviors.

By looking out for ADHD indicators such as careless attention to details, lack of focus and constant distraction, disorganization, impatience, restlessness, hyperactivity, and emotional instability among others, it is possible to spot ADHD in a child early on and catalyze treatment.

In Chapter 3, stories of parents caring for ADHD children took center stage. Moments of realization, struggles of keeping up with treatment and regimens, and eventual adaptation were shared in this chapter. Just like how I pretty much searched for a shoulder to cry on, a word to lean on, and a feeling that I was not going through alone while nursing my ADHD child, this chapter is that section of the book that gets down with you in the trenches.

As I shared my story and that of other parents with neurodiverse children, I believe you now possess the courage, motivation, and bravery required to nurture your ADHD child without resenting or neglecting. You found out that many parents have embraced the reality of parenting an ADHD child and taken control of helping their children as the occasion demands.

Chapter 4 describes the best way to manage your child's ADHD. Through a 3-Level management strategy, you see how to effectively manage your child's behaviors. The first level being strategies to make your child more focused, the second level being the strategies to keep your child motivated, and the third level being the strategies to keep your child educated. This chapter helps you to figure out how to synchronize all three levels to enhance your child's your child's lifestyle and create opportunities for fulfilling potentials.

In Chapter 5, you discovered the right way to reinforce the social skills of your child. Beyond the stigmatization that trails individuals who have ADHD, giving your child information about their condition dispels every form of stigma that might crush your child.

You found out that loving, accepting, and tutoring your child helps them find their feet and live above unsought and harsh opinions. By teaching your child how to deal with the rejection that comes with stigma, you prepare them for the future that they deserve in the world.

Finally, Chapter 6 elevates the importance of medication in coping with ADHD. You realized that leveraging groups that accommodate ADHD children and foster communities is inevitable in getting your child in tune with the world around them. More so, you recognized that therapy isn't only designed for your child but could also come in handy for you as a parent of an ADHD child.

The review of several pharmacological and non-pharmacological medications for ADHD children helps you to decide the best medication in favor of your child's growth. You familiarize yourself with the tenets of drug dosage, drug types, and drug detriment in this chapter. Thus, your new knowledge grants the ability to choose and select the right medicine relevant to your child's improvements. With the latest information delivered in this handbook, I believe you're now equipped to make the best decisions regarding the diagnosis, management, and treatment of your child.

Authors Note

Dear Reader,

I hope you enjoyed reading my book as much as I enjoyed writing it. Your feedback means the world to me, and I'd be incredibly grateful if you could take a moment to ***leave a review.***

The review will not only brighten my day but also help other potential readers discover the book.

So, please, share your thoughts, insights and feelings about this book. Thank you for your support.

Warmest wishes,

Sharon Daven

References

1. Pastor P, Reuben C, Duran C, Hawkins L. Association between diagnosed ADHD and selected characteristics among children aged 4–17 years: United States, 2011–2013. NCHS Data Brief. 2015;201:1–8.

2. Núñez-Jaramillo, L. Herrera-Solís, A. and Herrera-Morales, WV. 2021. ADHD: Reviewing the Causes and Evaluating Solutions. Journal of Personalized Medicine. 11(3):166.

3. Danielson, M.L. Bitsko, R.H. Ghandour, R.M. Holbrook, J.R. Kogan, M.D. Blumberg, S.J. (2016). Prevalence of parent-reported ADHD diagnosis and associated treatment among U.S. children and adolescents. In J Clin Child Adolescent Psychol. (2018).

4. World population review. 2023. ADHD by country 2023. https://worldpopulationreview.com/country-rankings/adhd-rates-by-country

5. American Psychiatric Association. (1994). Diagnostic and statistical manual of mental disorders (4th ed.). Washington DC.

6. American Psychiatric Association. 2013. Diagnostic and statistical manual of mental disorders fifth edition.

7. Hallowell, E.M. & J.J. Ratey (2006), Delivered from distraction: Getting the most out of life with Attention Deficit Disorder. New York: Ballantine Books.

8. Armstrong, T. (2003). Attention Deficit Hyperactivity Disorder in children: one consequence of the rise of technology and demise of play. In Shama Olfman (ed.) All Work and No Play…How Eductional Reforms Are Harming Our Prescholars. Westport Ct.: Praeger, pp. 161-16.

9. Kahn, R.S., Khoury, J., Nicholas, W.C., & Lanphear, B.P. (2003). Role of dopamine transporter genotype and maternal prenatal smoking in childhood hyperactive-impulsive, inattentive, and oppositional behaviors. J. Pediatrics 143; pp. 104-110.

10. First Psychology. Understanding ADHD in children and adults. www.firstpsychology.co.uk.

11. Wender, E. H. (2002) Editorial: Attention-Deficit/Hyperactivity Disorder: Is it common? Is it overtreated? Archives of Pediatric and Adolescent Medicine. 156, 209-210.

12. Morris-Rosendahl DJ. 2020. Neurodevelopmental disorders—the history and future of a diagnostic concept. Dialogues Clin Neurosci. 22(1)

13. IACAPAP Textbook of Child and Adolescent Mental Health

14. First Psychology. Understanding ADHD in children and adult. www.firstpsychology.co.uk

15. Thomas, E. B. (2017). Exaggerated Emotions: How and Why ADHD Triggers Intense Feelings. Retrieved from

https://www.additudemag.com/slideshows/adhd-emotions-understanding-intense-feelings/

16. Lite, Jordan. (2013). A real mom's story: raising a child with ADHD. In Today Health and Wellness. https://www.today.com/health/real-moms-story-raising-child-adhd-1123149

17. Jackson, Carrie. (2023). Best todo apps for ADHD symptoms: the top 6. Retrieved from https://www.joonapp.io/post/best-todo-app-for-adhd

18. https://www.healthline.com/health/mental-health/how-to-stay-focused#avoid-multitasking

19. Repantis, D. Bovy, L. Ohla, K. Kühn, S. & Dresler, M. (2021). Cognitive enhancement effects of stimulants: a randomized controlled trial testing methylphenidate, modafinil, and caffeine. In National Library of Medicine. 238(2). 441-451

20. ADHD experts at ADDitude. 10 things you should never say to your child.

21. American Psychological Association. Understanding Psychotherapy and how it works. Retrieved from https://www.cdc.gov/ncbddd/adhd/treatment.html#:~:text=Several%20different%20types%20of%20medications, taking%20these%20fast%2Dacting%20medications.

22. Centers for disease and control and prevention. Attention Deficit / Hyperactivity Disorder (ADHD) Treatment

23. Greenhill, L. Swanson, J. Hechtman, L. et al (2019). Trajectories of growth associated with long-term stimulant medication in the multimodal treatment study of Attention –Deficit/Hyperactivity Disorder. Journal of the American Academy if Child and Adolescent Pst=ychiatry, S0890-8567(19).

24. Fewell, R. & Deutscher, B. (2002). Attention Deficit Hyperactivity Disorder in very young children: early signs and interventions. Inf Young Children. 14(3), 24-32.